M Mosby
Year Book
Dedicated to Publishing Excellence

Publisher: George Stamathis
Editor-in-Chief: Anne S. Patterson
Assistant Editor: Dana Battaglia
Project Manager: Patricia Tannian
Production Editor: Ann E. Rogers
Designer: David Zielinski

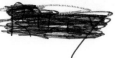

W9-CFH-015

Copyright © 1993 by Mosby-Year Book, Inc.
A Mosby imprint of Mosby-Year Book, Inc.

All rights reserved. No part of this publication may be reproduced, stored in a retrieval system, or transmitted, in any form or by any means, electronic, mechanical, photocopying, recording, or otherwise, without prior written permission from the publisher.

Permission to photocopy or reproduce solely for internal or personal use is permitted for libraries or other users registered with the Copyright Clearance Center, provided that the base fee of $4.00 per chapter plus $.10 per page is paid directly to the Copyright Clearance Center, 27 Congress Street, Salem, MA 01970. This consent does not extend to other kinds of copying, such as copying for general distribution, for advertising or promotional purposes, for creating new collected works, or for resale.

Printed in the United States of America

Mosby-Year Book, Inc.
11830 Westline Industrial Drive
St. Louis, Missouri 63146

Library of Congress Cataloging in Publication Data

Practical alimentary tract radiology / edited by Alexander R.
 Margulis, H. Joachim Burhenne.
      p.   cm.
    Based on: Alimentary tract radiology. 4th ed. 1989.
    Includes index.
    ISBN 0-8016-3133-5
    1. Gastrointestinal system—Radiography.   I. Margulis, Alexander
 R.   II. Burhenne, H. Joachim (Hans Joachim), 1925-
 III. Alimentary tract radiology.
      [DNLM: 1. Digestive System—radiography.   WI 141 P8944]
 RC804.R6P73 1992
 616.3'307572—dc20
 DNLM/DLC   92-18766
 for Library of Congress   CIP

93 94 95 96 97 CL/MV 9 8 7 6 5 4 3 2 1

Practical Alimentary Tract Radiology

Edited by

Alexander R. Margulis, M.D.

Professor, Department of Radiology
Associate Chancellor–Special Projects
University of California, San Francisco
San Francisco, California

H. Joachim Burhenne, M.D., FRCP(C), FFRRCSI (Hon.)

Professor, Department of Radiology
University of British Columbia
Vancouver General Hospital
Vancouver, British Columbia, Canada

*With **1089** illustrations*

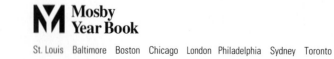
Mosby
Year Book

St. Louis Baltimore Boston Chicago London Philadelphia Sydney Toronto